I0829590

Music Credits:
"Chicken Fat" also known as "The Youth Fitness Song"
Performed by Robert Preston | Written by Meredith Wilson

Acknowledgements:
A special thanks to Noelle, Erica, and Eric.

To Sing-A-Long, Please Visit Our Website:

ChickenFatKids.com

Disclaimer:
Not all exercises are suitable for everyone and this or any other exercise program may result in injury. Any user of this exercise program assumes the risk of injury resulting from performing the exercises. To reduce the risk of injury, consult your doctor before beginning this exercise program. The instructions and advice presented are not intended as a substitute for medical counseling. The creators, producers and distributers of this program disclaim any liabilities in connection with exercise and advice herein.

CHICKEN FAT

(To sing-a-long, visit ChickenFatKids.com)

created by SCOTT DRAYER

illustrated by MATT HUSON

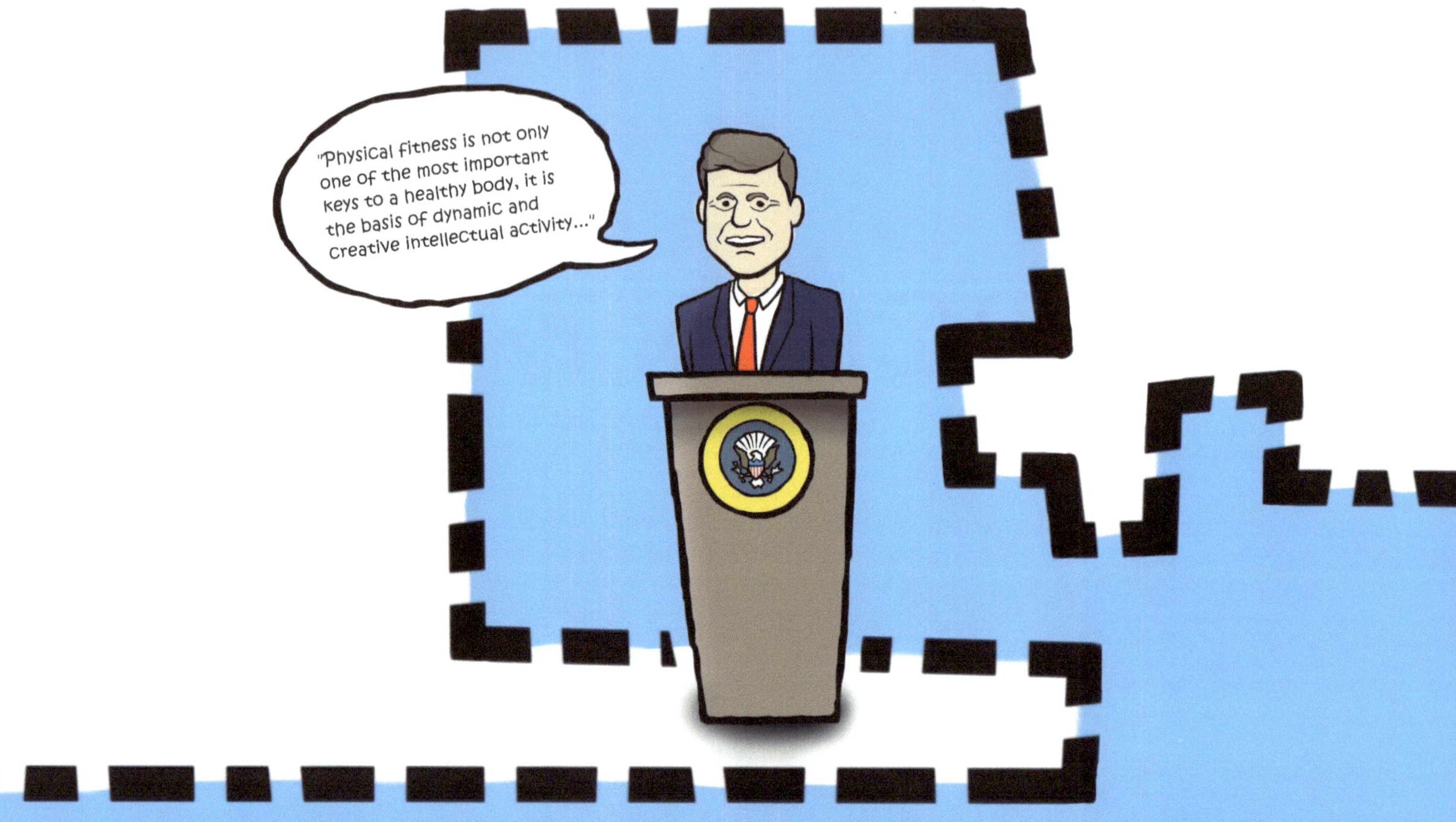

In the 1960's, President John F. Kennedy announced that the President's Council on Physical Fitness was beginning a physical fitness program for schools. Inspired by the idea, Meredith Wilson - composer of " The Music Man", "The Unsinkable Molly Brown", and "Till There Was You", a song which was later recorded by the Beatles - immediately wrote "Chicken Fat" as his contribution to the Kennedy fitness program. Since it's beginning "Chicken Fat" has been one of the most popular youth fitness programs in the nation. This book has been created in the spirit of fitness and fun for all!

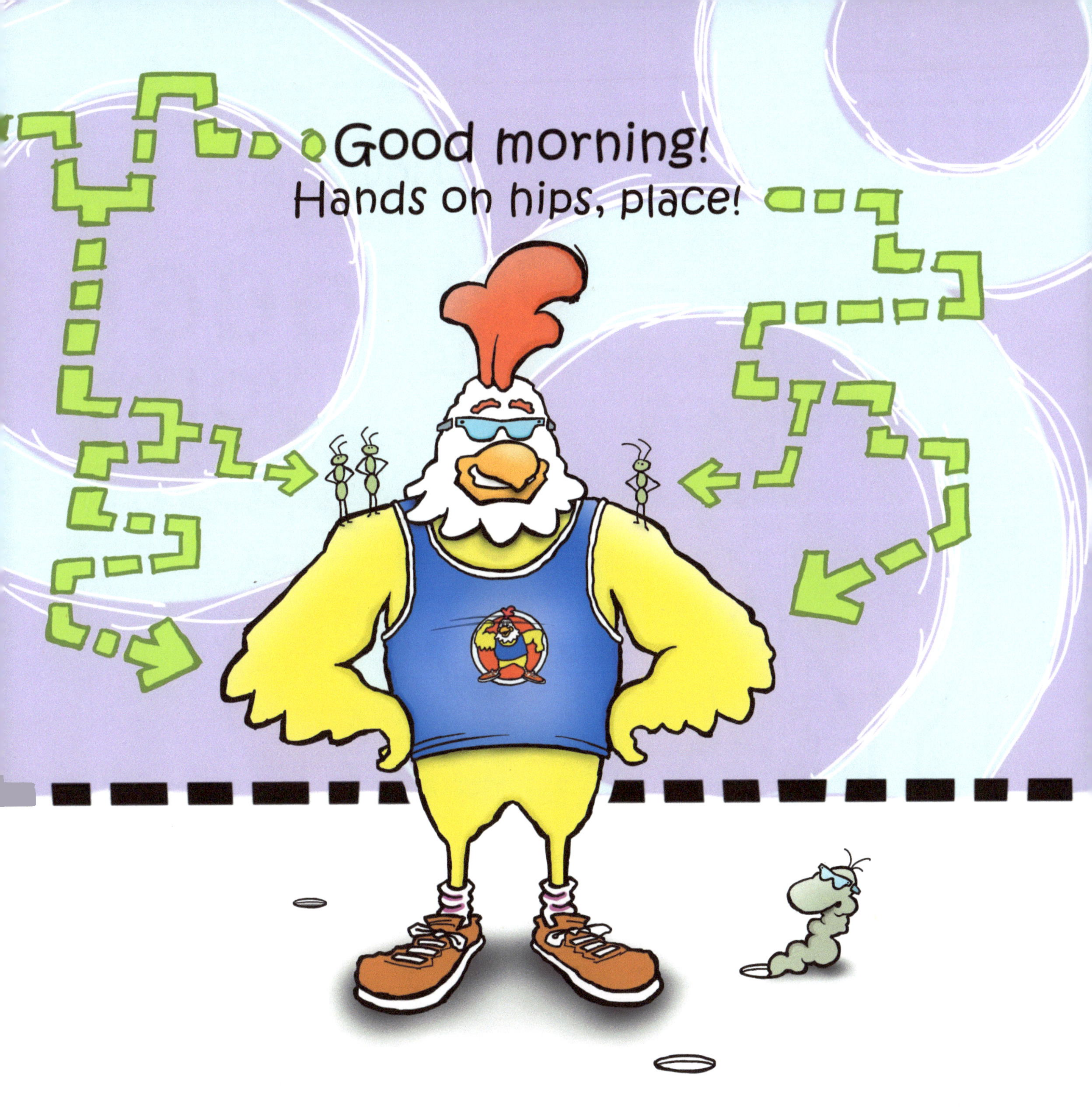

Good morning!
Hands on hips, place!

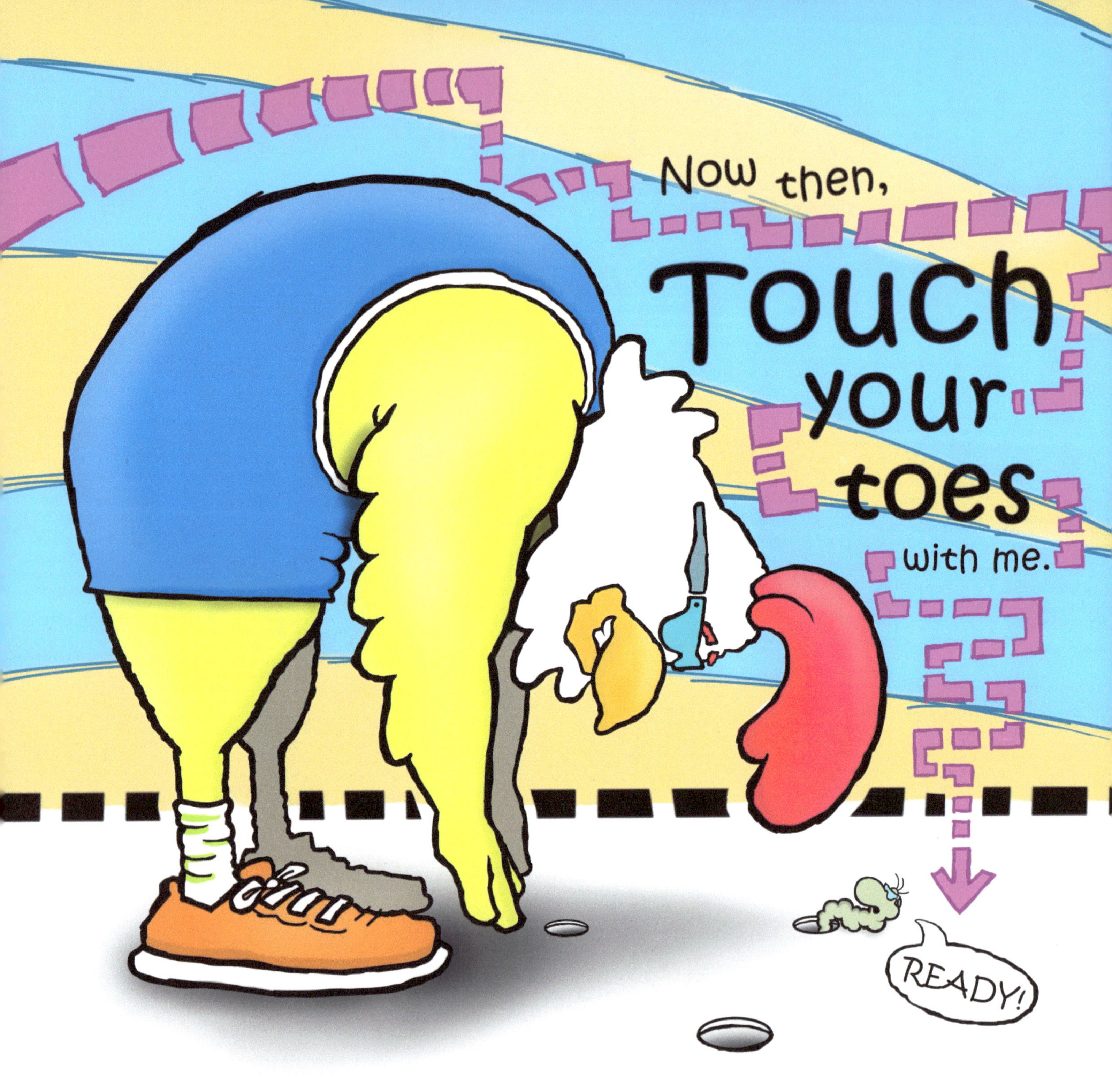

Now then,
Touch
your
toes
with me.
READY!

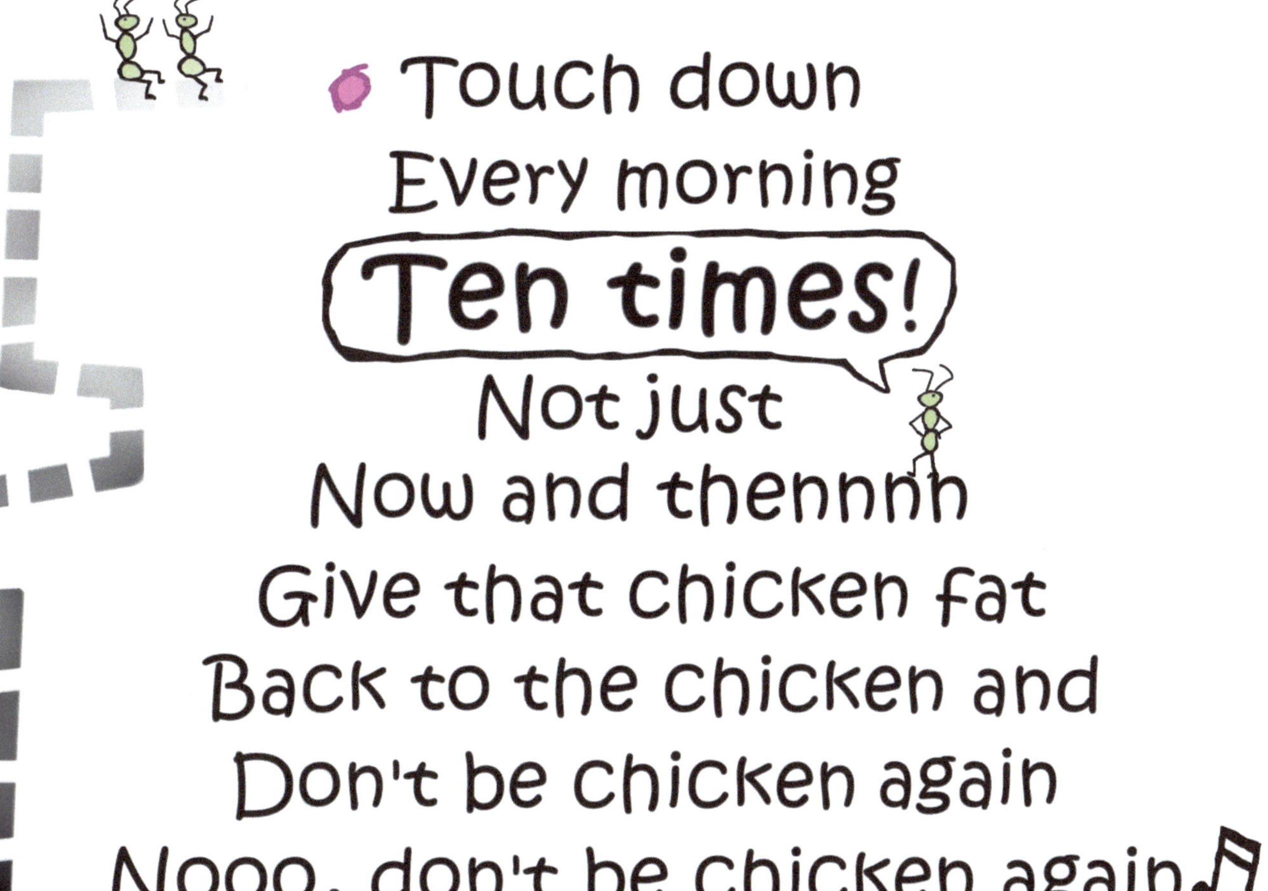

Touch down
Every morning
Ten times!
Not just
Now and thennnn
Give that chicken fat
Back to the chicken and
Don't be chicken again
Nooo, don't be chicken again

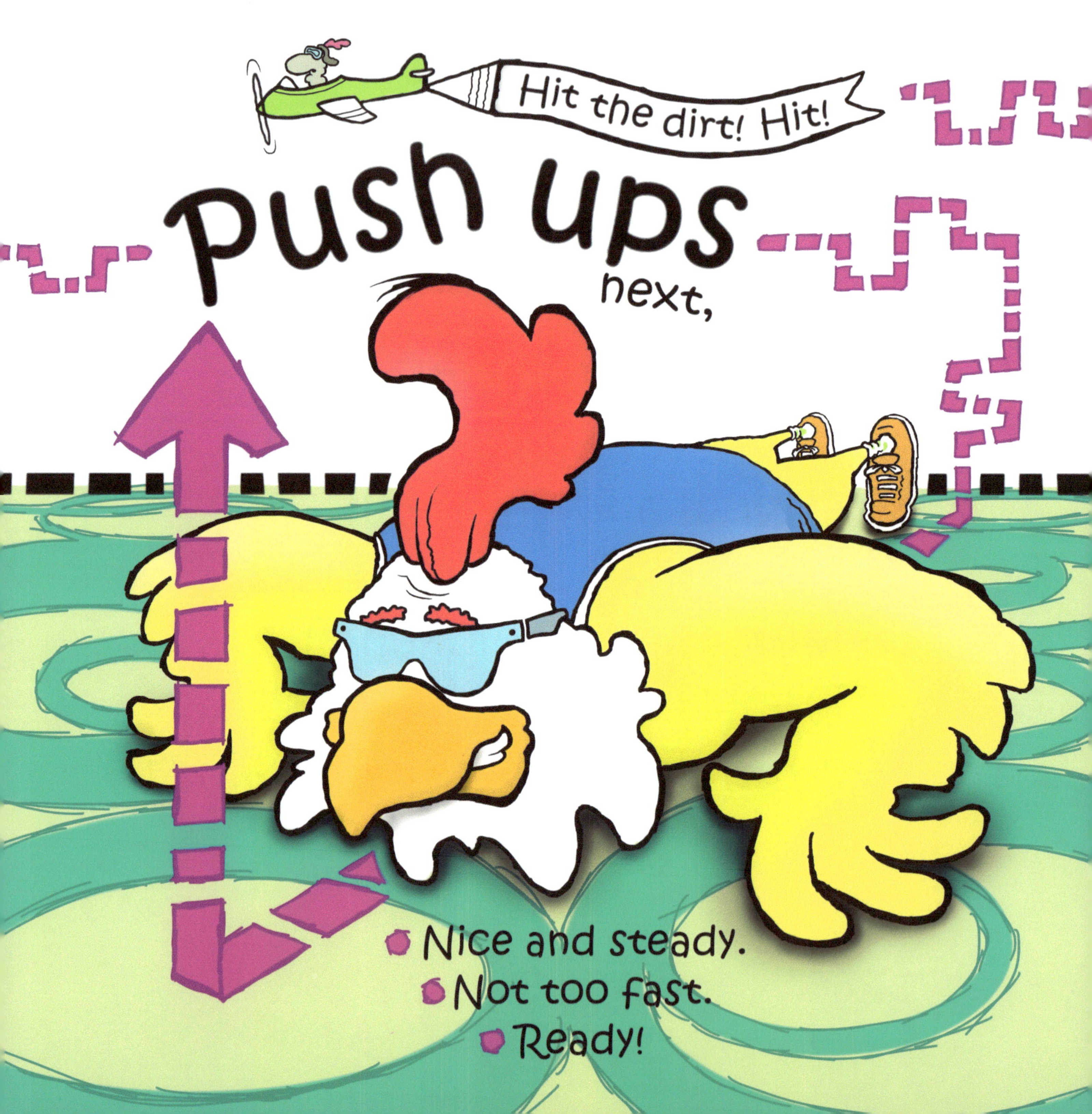
Hit the dirt! Hit!
Push ups
next,
Nice and steady.
Not too fast.
Ready!

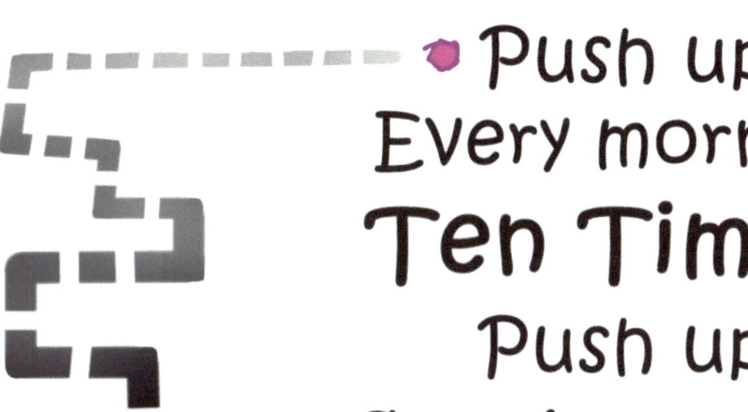

Push up
Every morning
Ten Times!
Push up,
Starting lowww.
Once more on the rise
Nuts to the flabby guys,
Go, you chicken fat, go awayyy
Go, you chicken fat, go!

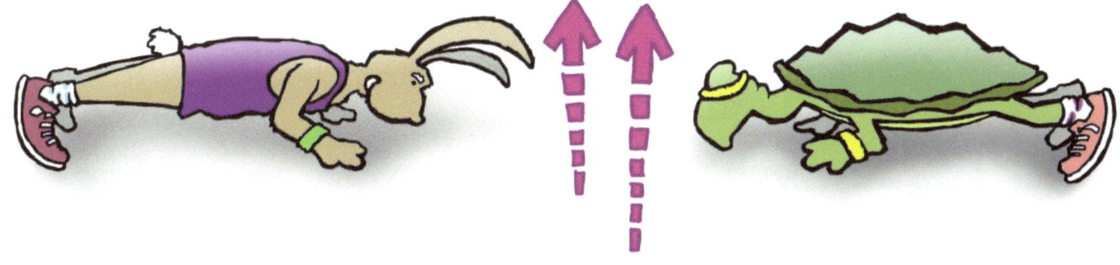

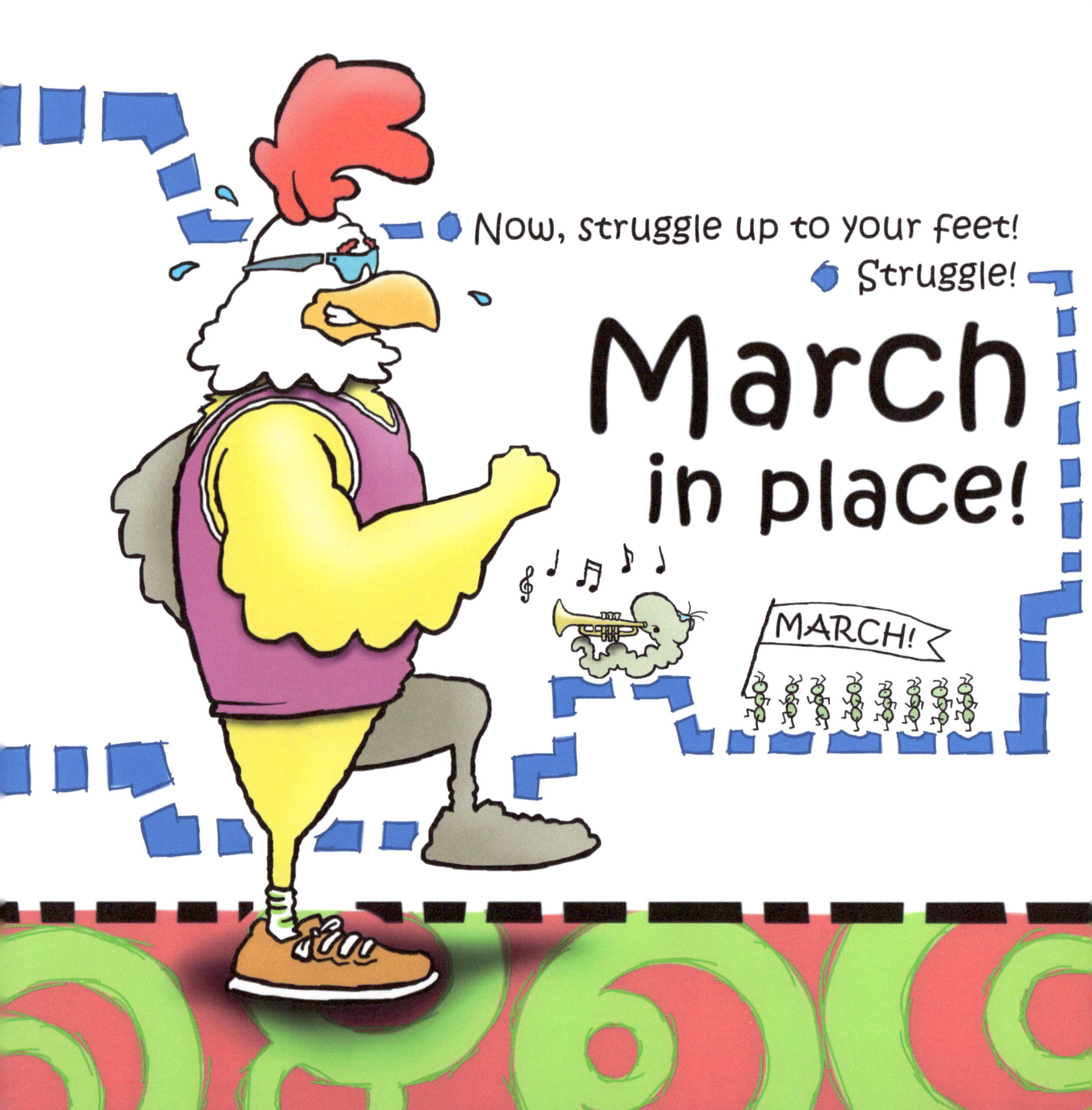

Now, struggle up to your feet!
Struggle!
March
in place!
MARCH!

Left! Left! Left! Left!
Left a good pound and a quarter.
Was it right, right that it should be left?
Yes left! Left! Left! Left!
Left a good pound and a quarter.
It was right, right that it should be left!

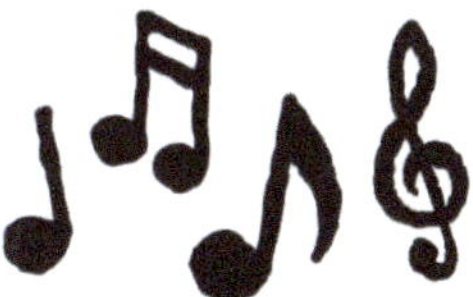

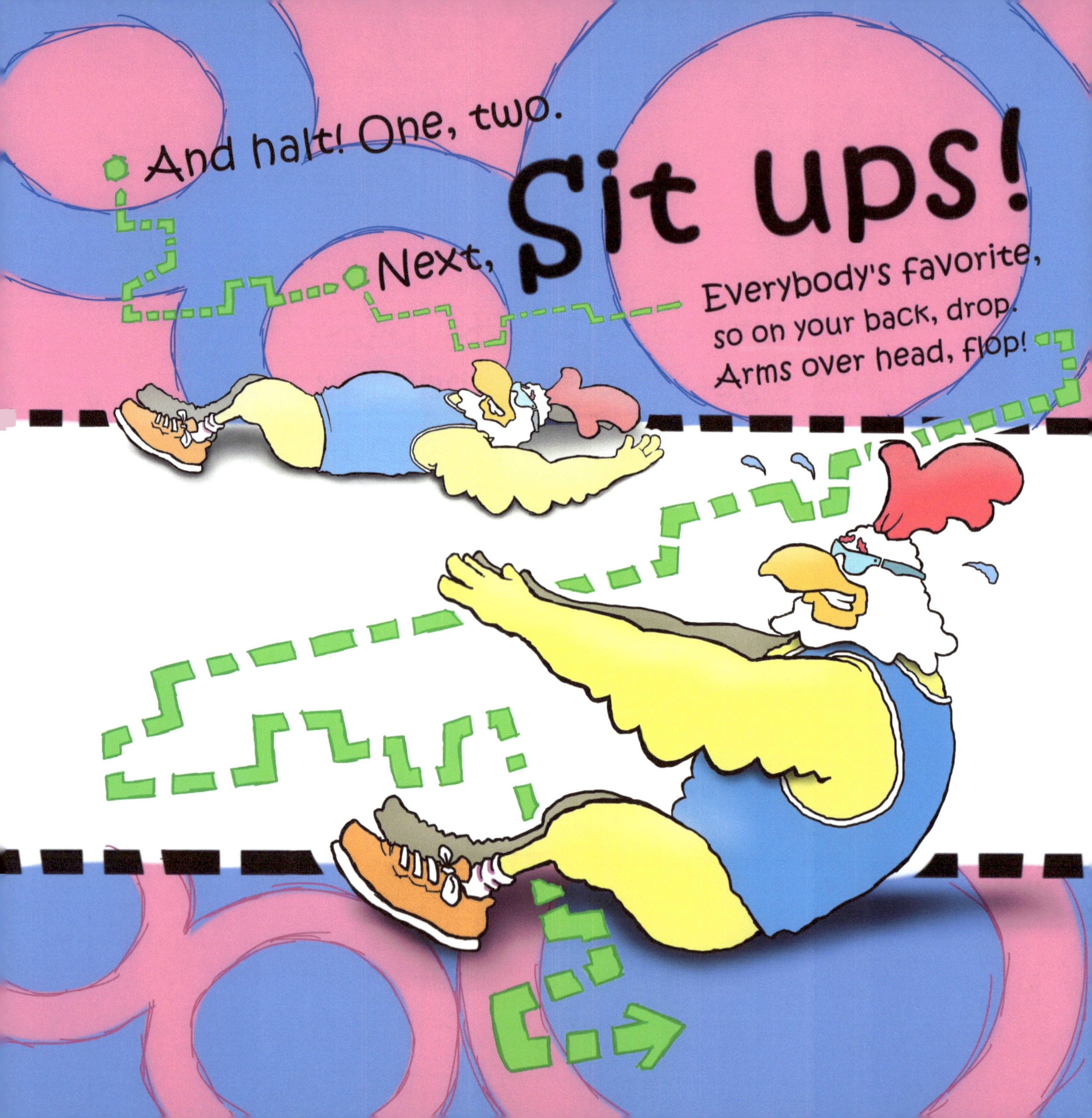

And halt! One, two.
Next, Sit ups!
Everybody's favorite,
so on your back, drop.
Arms over head, flop!

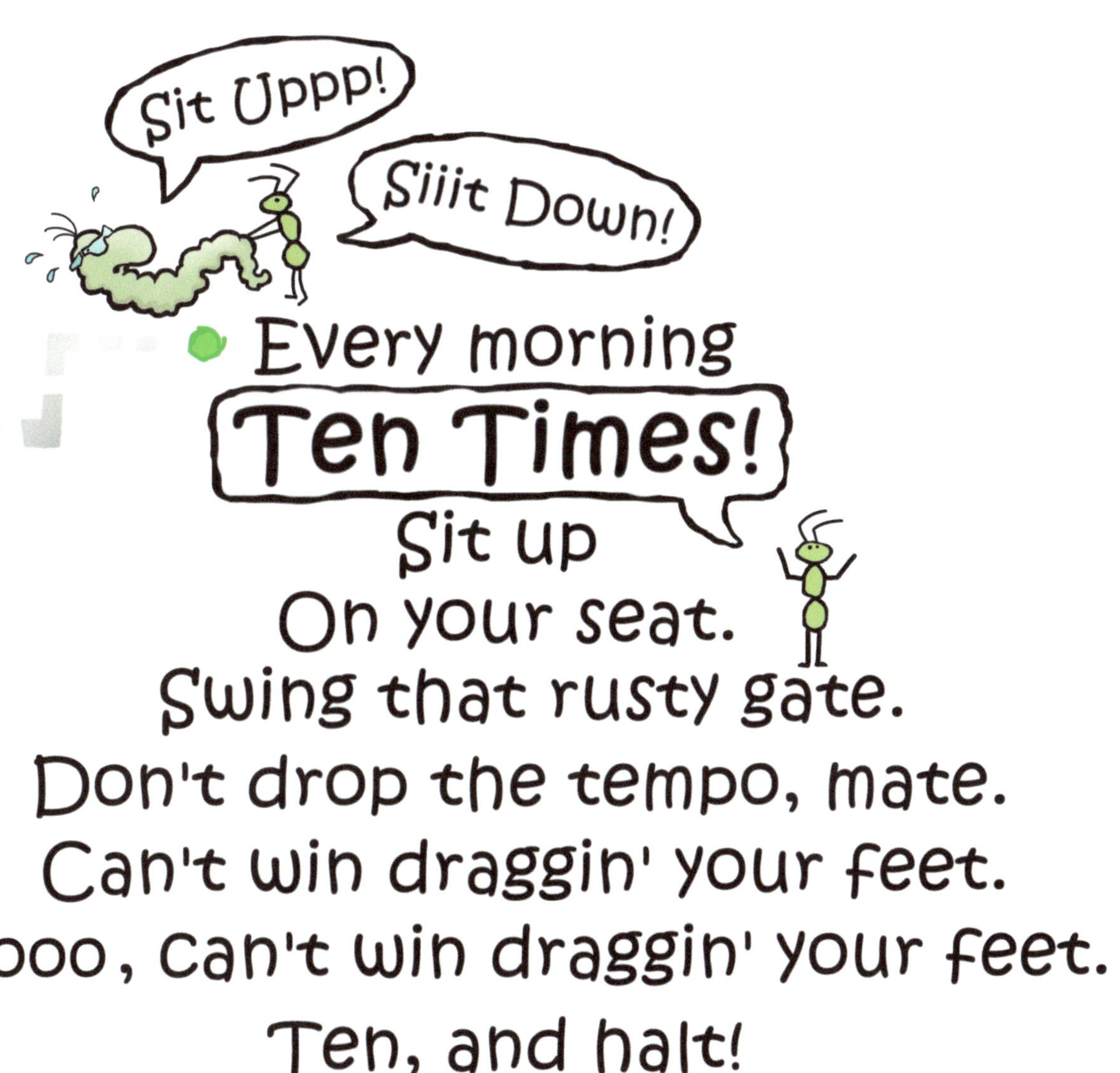

Every morning
Sit up
On your seat.
Swing that rusty gate.
Don't drop the tempo, mate.
Can't win draggin' your feet.
Nooo, can't win draggin' your feet.
Ten, and halt!

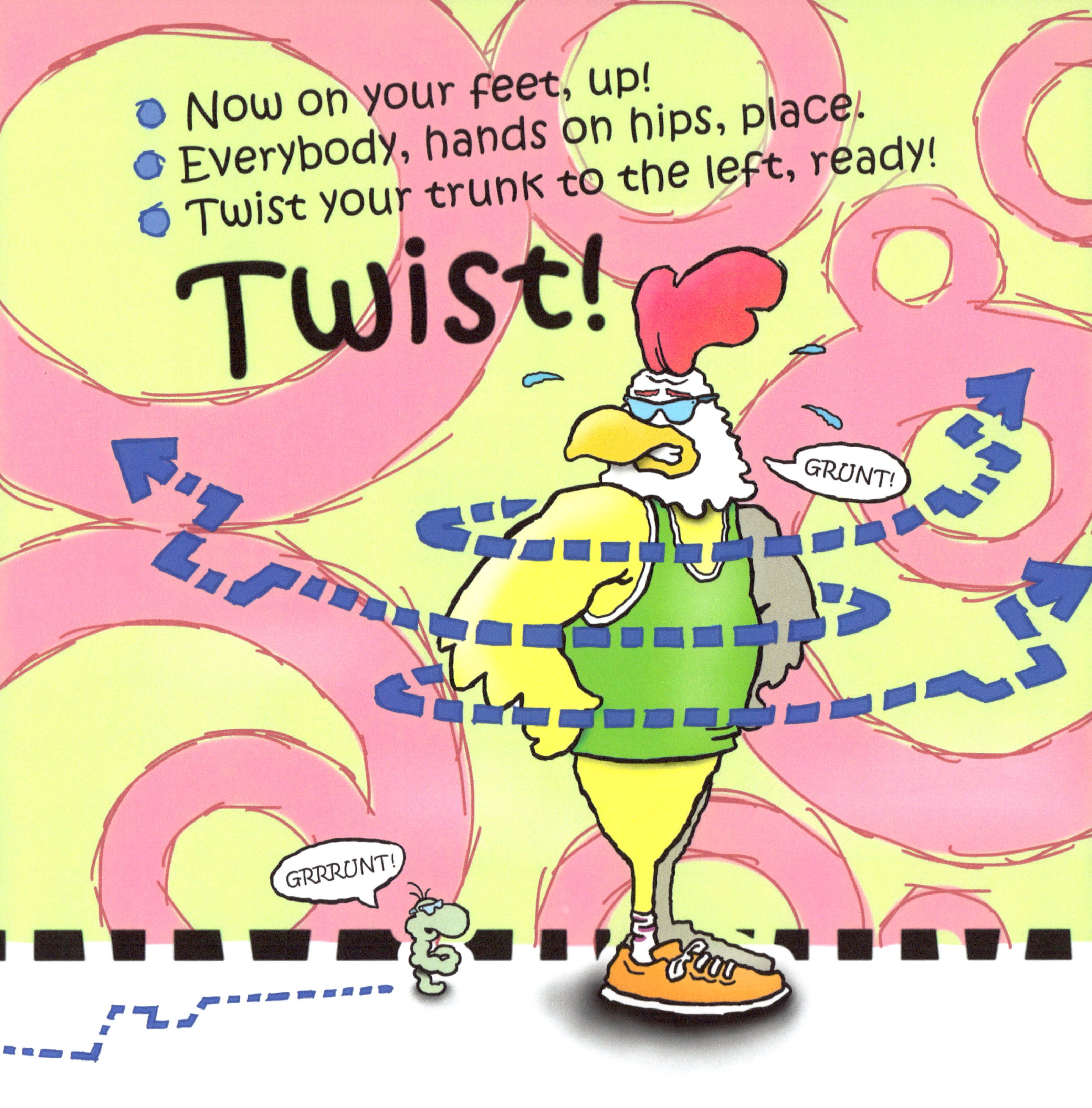

Now on your feet, up!
Everybody, hands on hips, place.
Twist your trunk to the left, ready!
Twist!
GRUNT!
GRRRUNT!

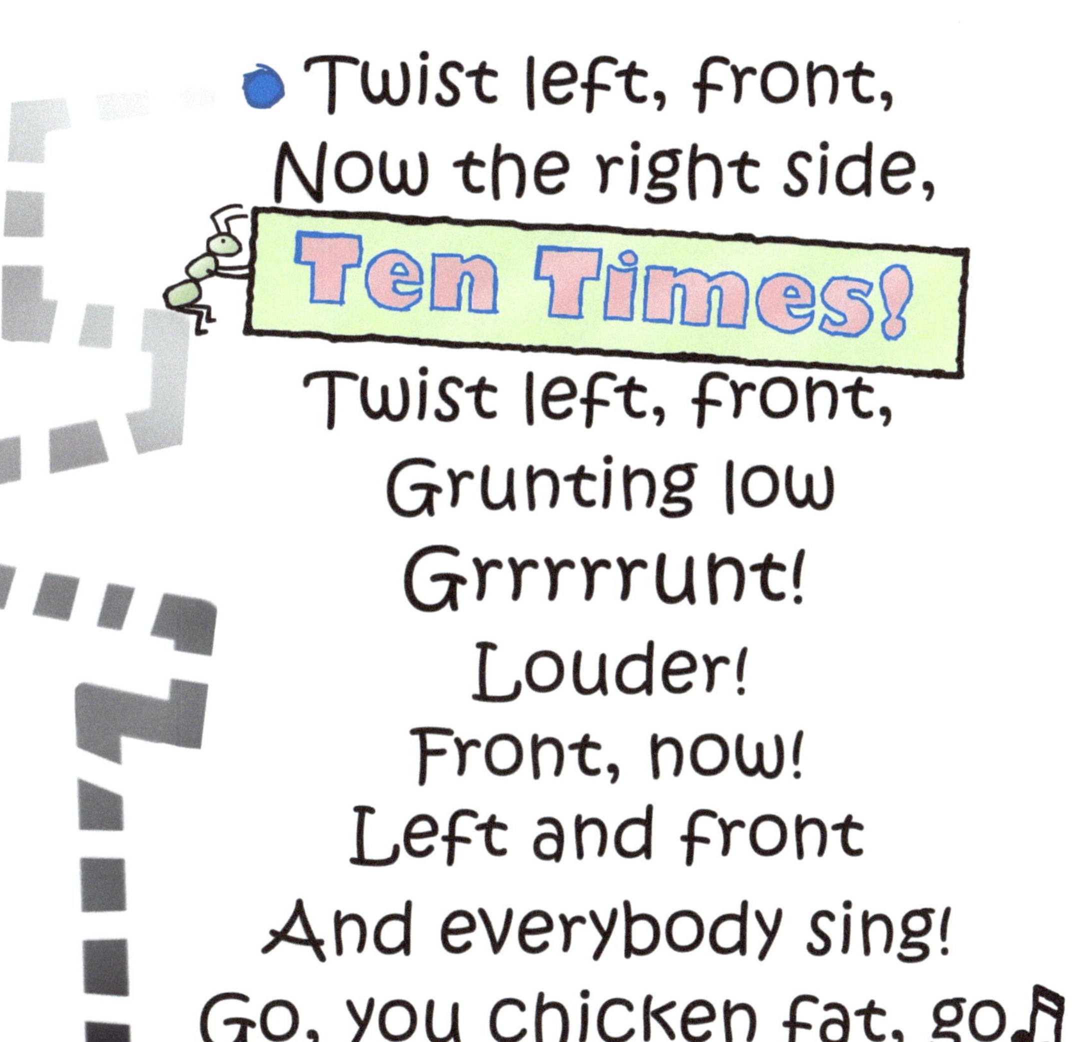
Twist left, front,
Now the right side,
Ten Times!
Twist left, front,
Grunting low
Grrrrunt!
Louder!
Front, now!
Left and front
And everybody sing!
Go, you chicken fat, go♫

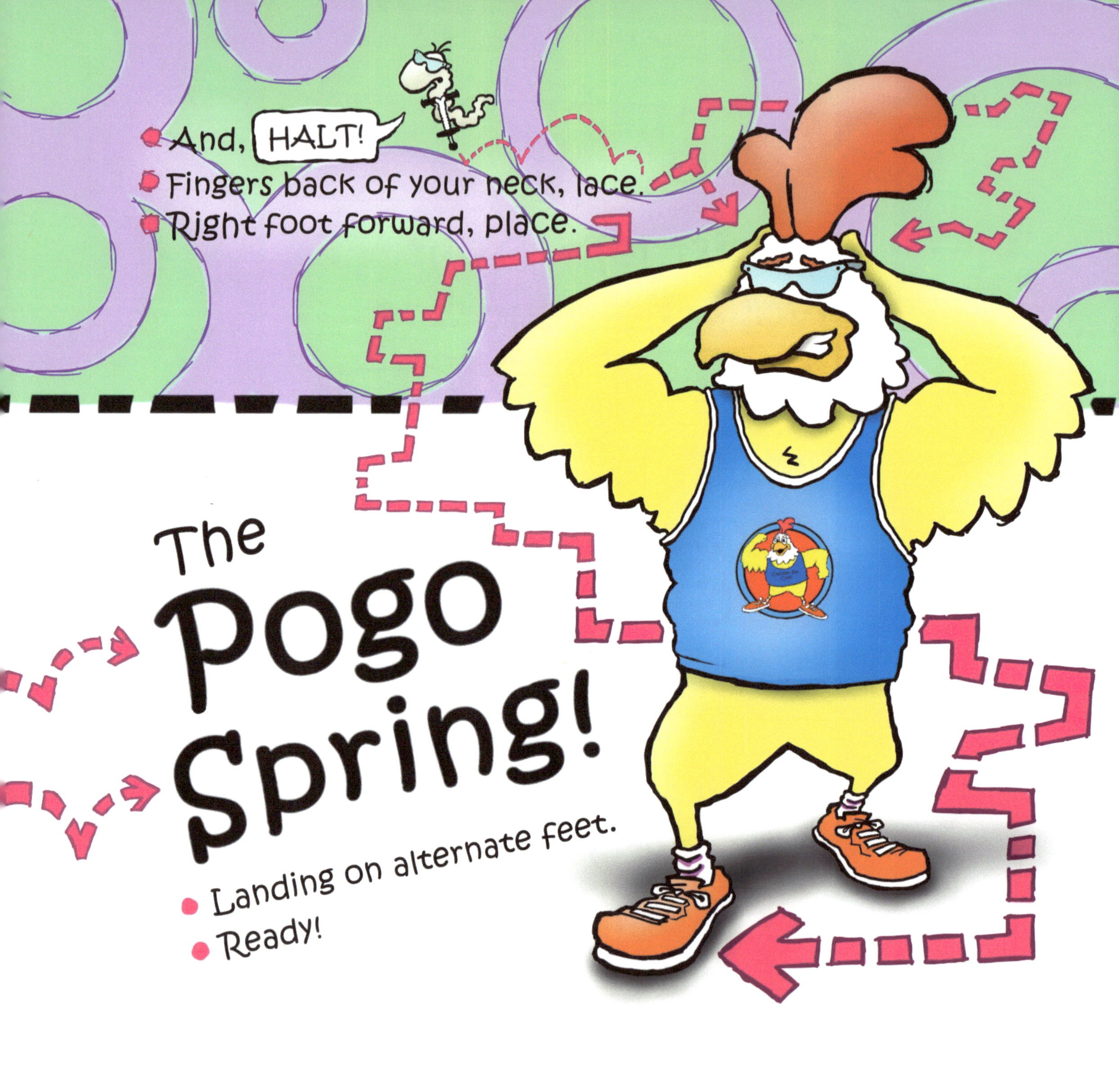
And, HALT!
Fingers back of your neck, lace.
Right foot forward, place.

The
Pogo
Spring!

Landing on alternate feet.
Ready!

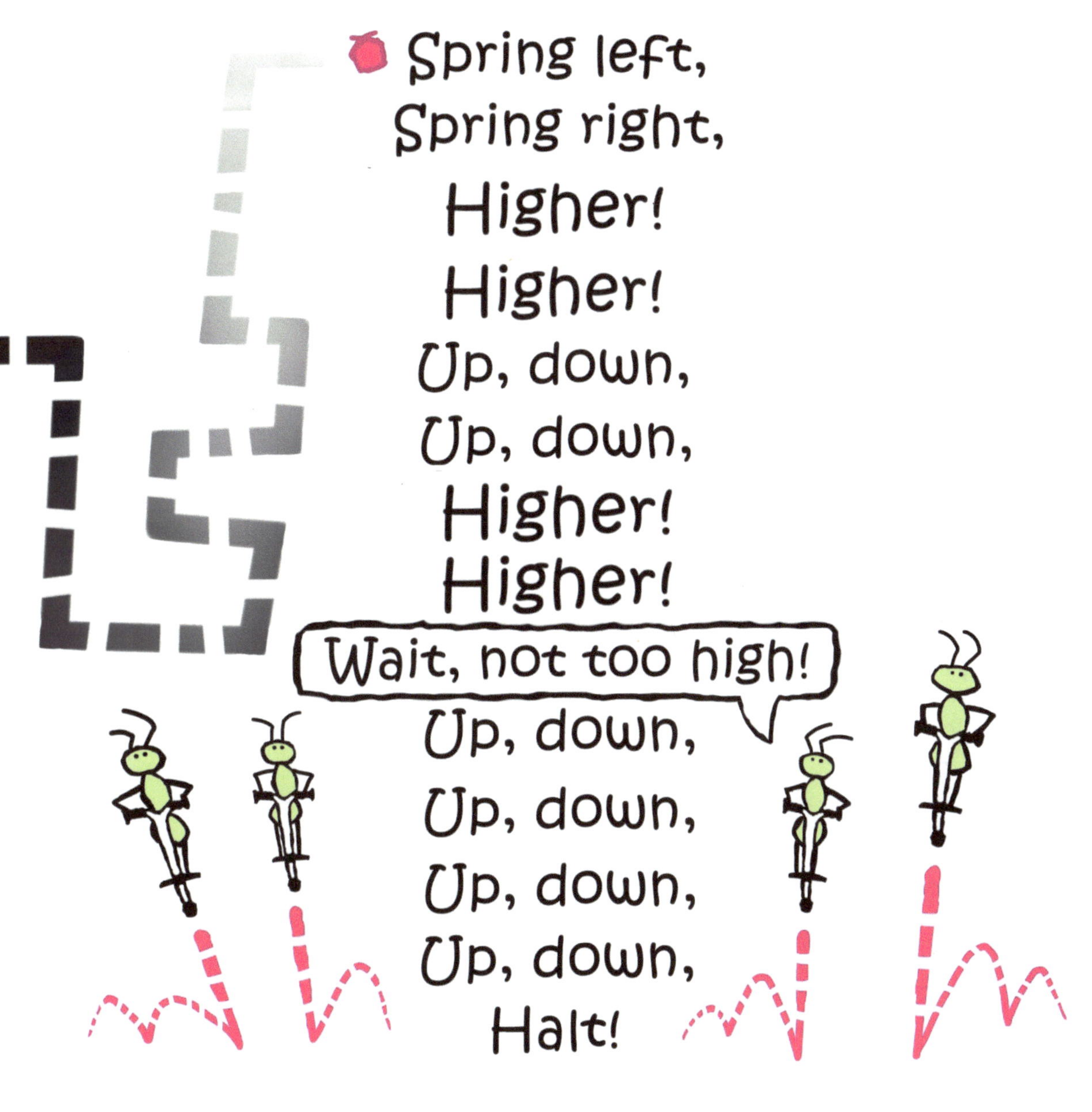
Spring left,
Spring right,
Higher!
Higher!
Up, down,
Up, down,
Higher!
Higher!
Wait, not too high!
Up, down,
Up, down,
Up, down,
Up, down,
Halt!

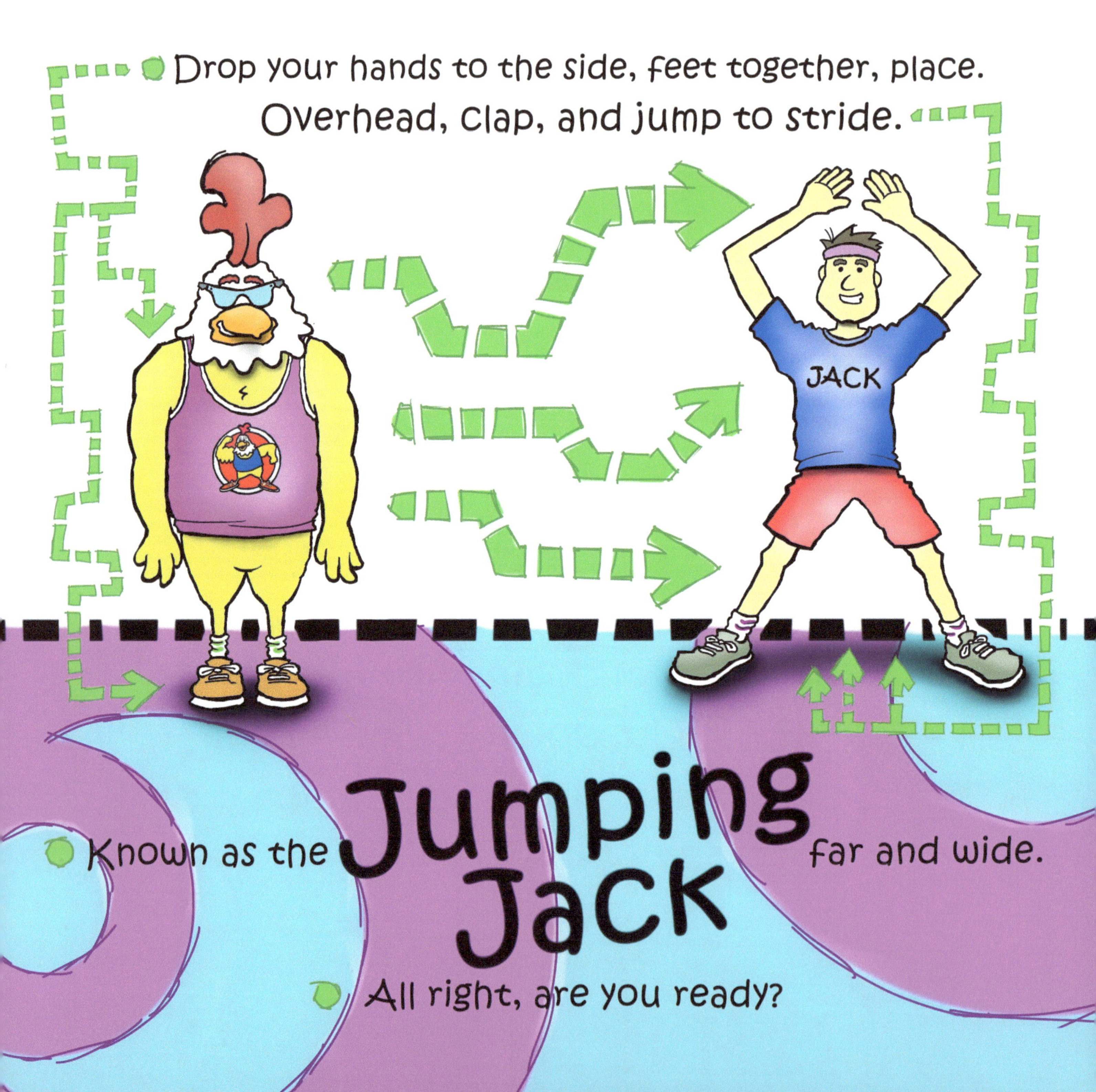

Drop your hands to the side, feet together, place.
Overhead, clap, and jump to stride.

JACK

Known as the Jumping Jack far and wide.

All right, are you ready?

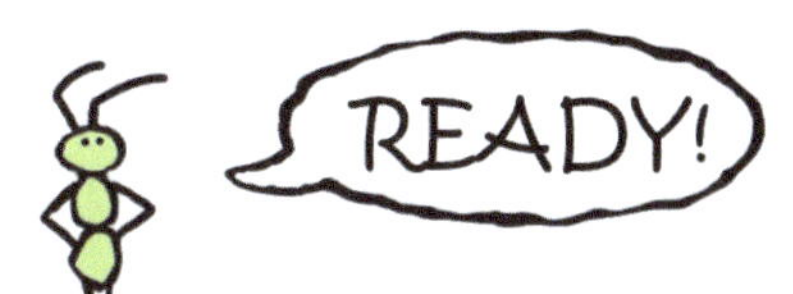

Jump, two! Clap, two!
Clap, two! Clap, slap!
Clap, slap! Clap, slap!
Jump, two! Jump, two!
Jump, it's good for you.
Three more is all we do.
Jump, two!
And...halt and sing!
Go, you chicken fat, gooo!!!

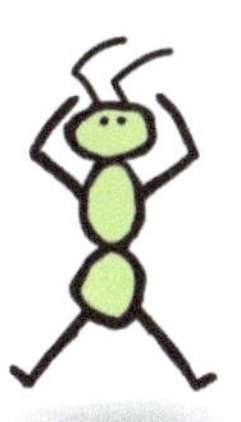
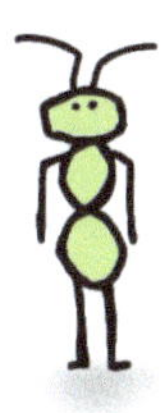
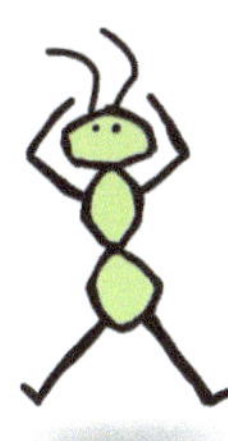

March in place!

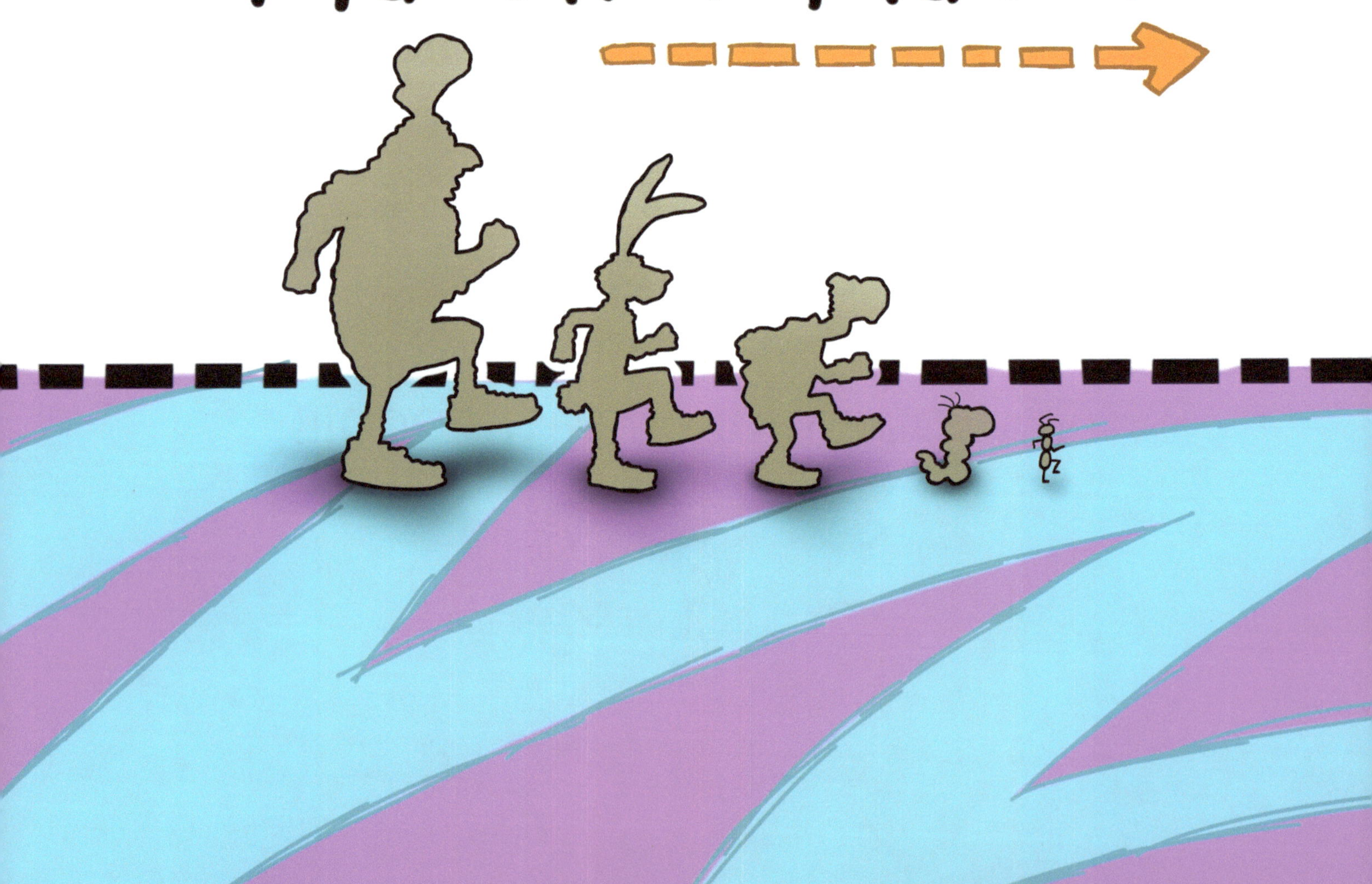

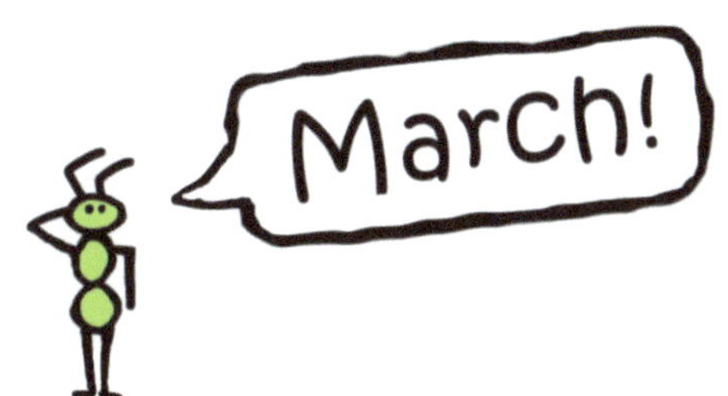

Left! Left! Left! Left!
Left a good pound and a quarter.
Was it right, right that it should be left?
Yes left! Left! Left! Left!
It was right, right left, and Halt, one two.

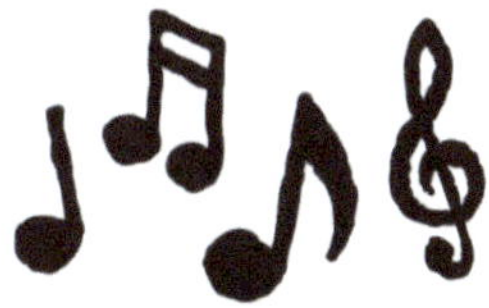

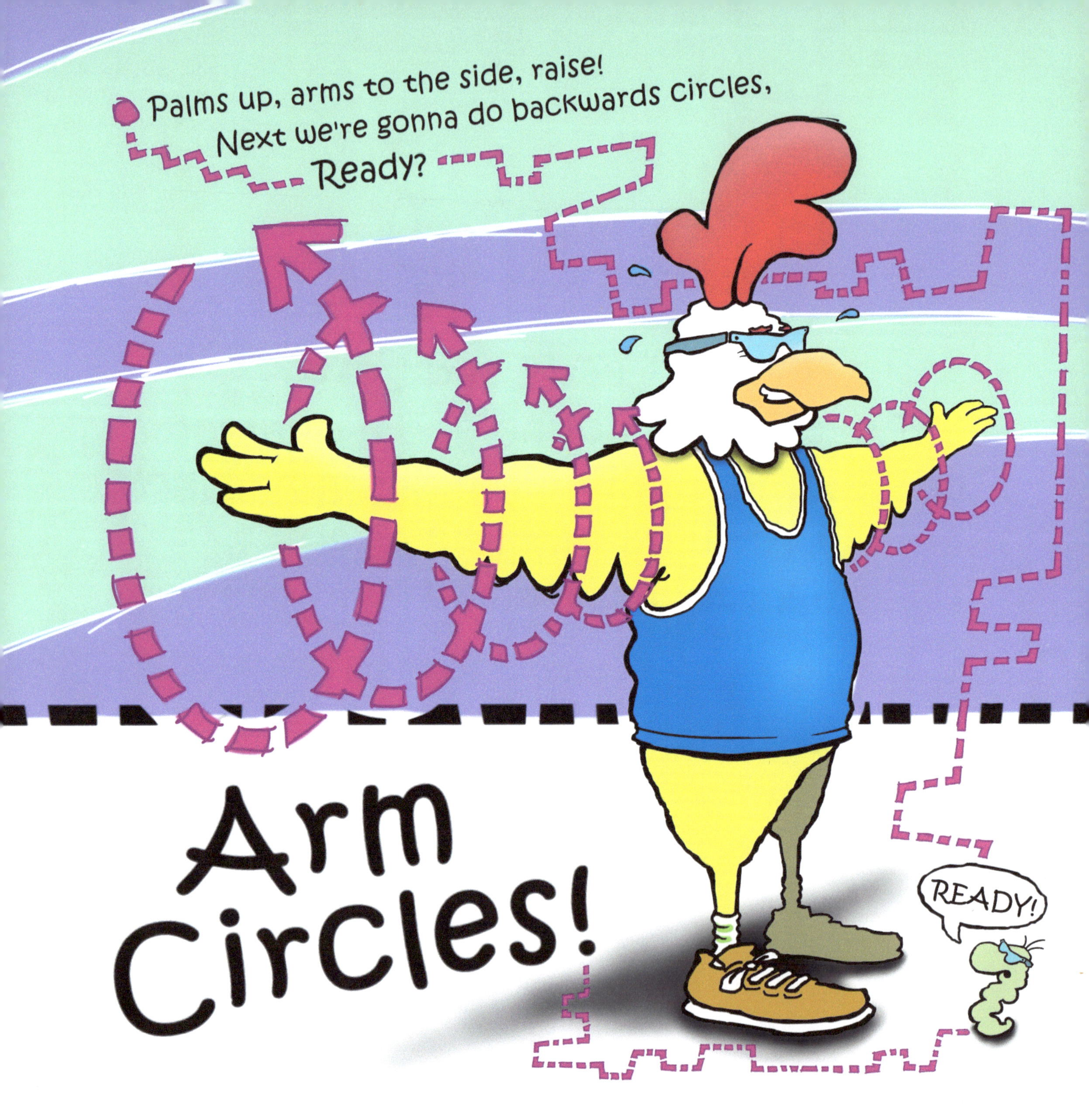

Palms up, arms to the side, raise!
Next we're gonna do backwards circles,
Ready?
Arm Circles!
READY!

Circle round, round, round
Back and around, back and around.
Back and around, back and around.
And back and around, and reverse.
And around, Front and around.
Front and around, front and around.
Front and around, and halt.

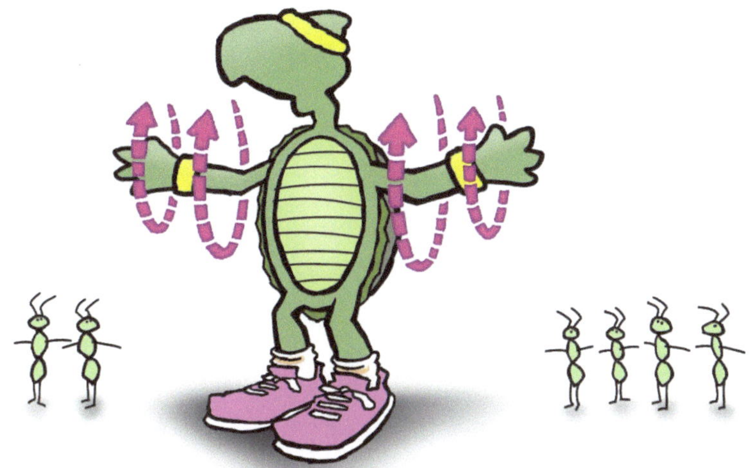

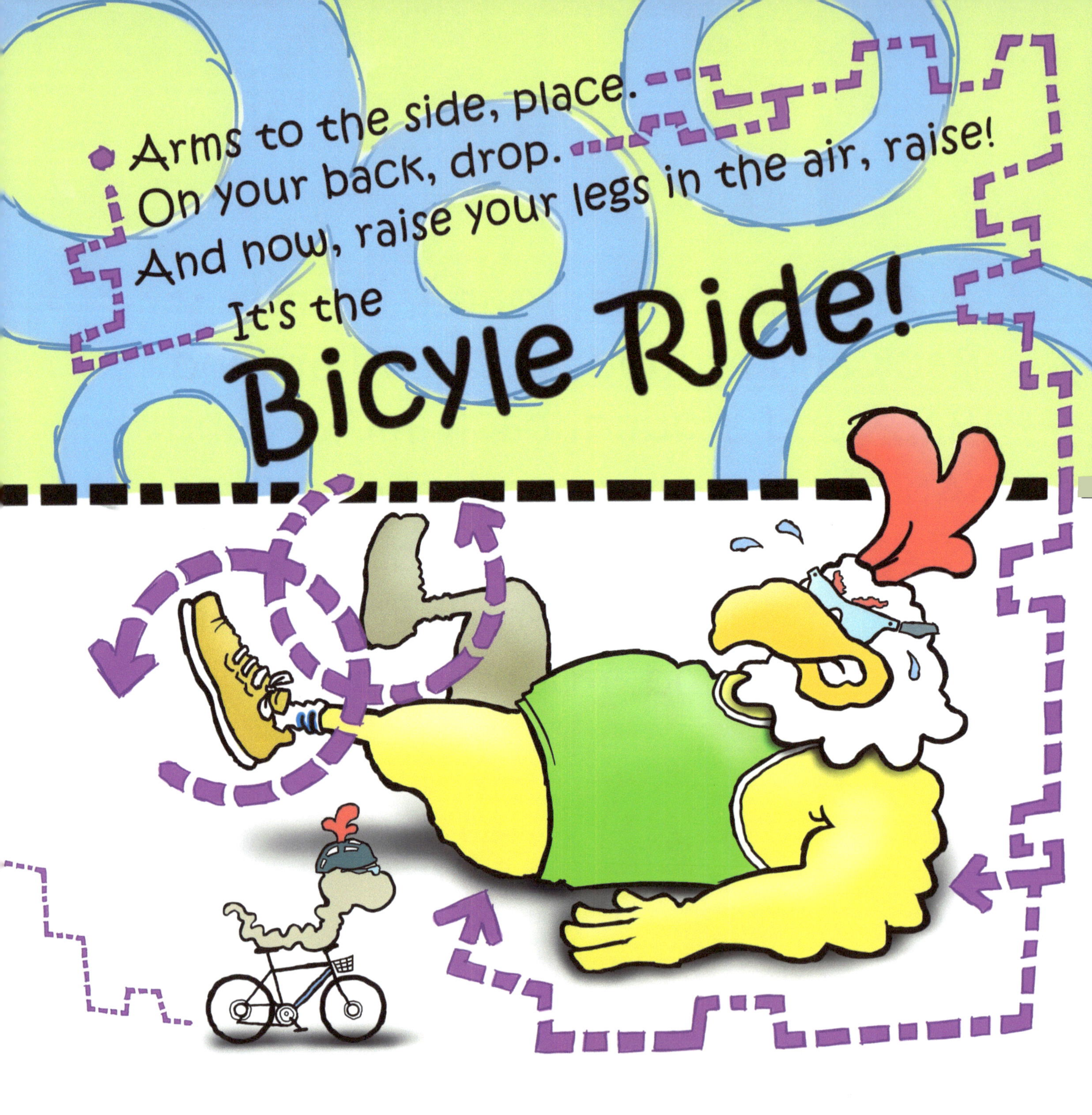

Arms to the side, place.
On your back, drop.
And now, raise your legs in the air, raise!
It's the
Bicyle Ride!

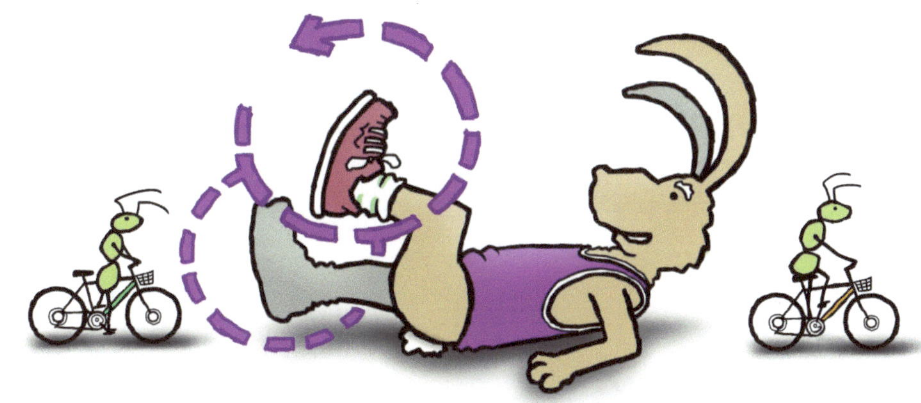

And, pump, pump, pump, pump,
Pump, pump, pump, pump,
Pump, pump, pump, pump,
Pump, pump, and...

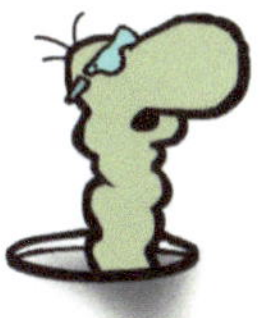

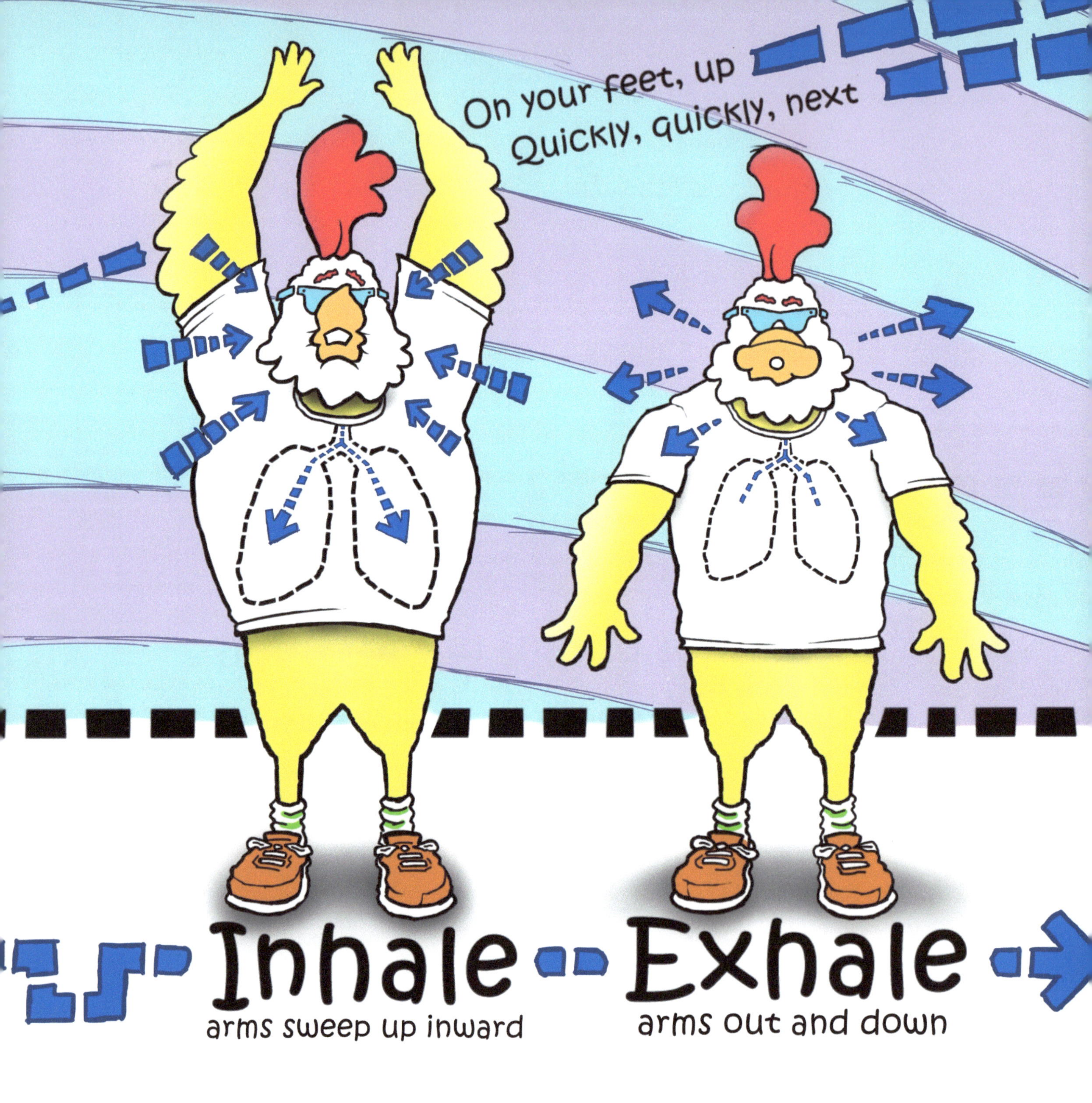

On your feet, up
Quickly, quickly, next
Inhale
arms sweep up inward
Exhale
arms out and down

Inhale slow
Every morning
Exhale, clear down.
Inhale, take the air!
Down and around and inhale.
Grab that oxygen,
Exhale and try again!
You're not getting your share.
No, you're not getting your share!

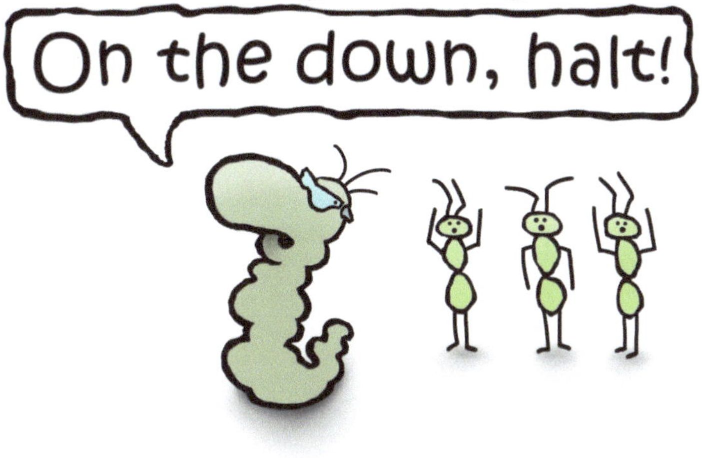

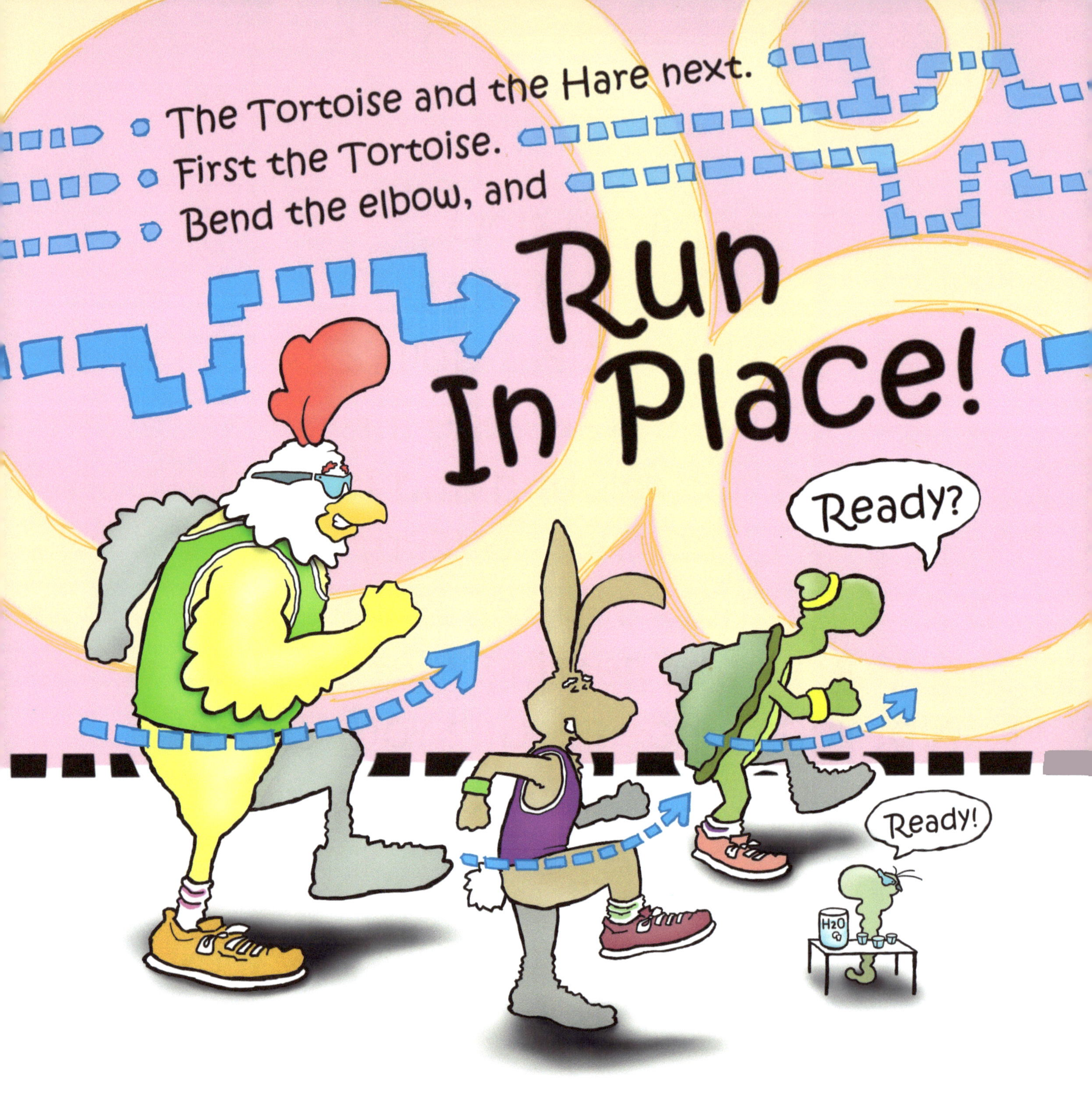

The Tortoise and the Hare next.
First the Tortoise.
Bend the elbow, and
Run In Place!
Ready?
Ready!
H2O

Running,
Like a tortoise,
Too far, and too slow.
Now double up, ready!
Run two three four,
Run two three four,
Run two three four,
Run two three four,
Go you chicken fat,
Go away!
Everybody sing!
Go, you chicken fat, go!

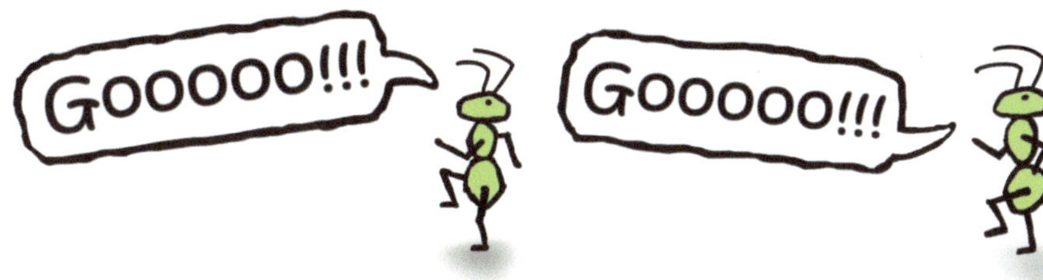

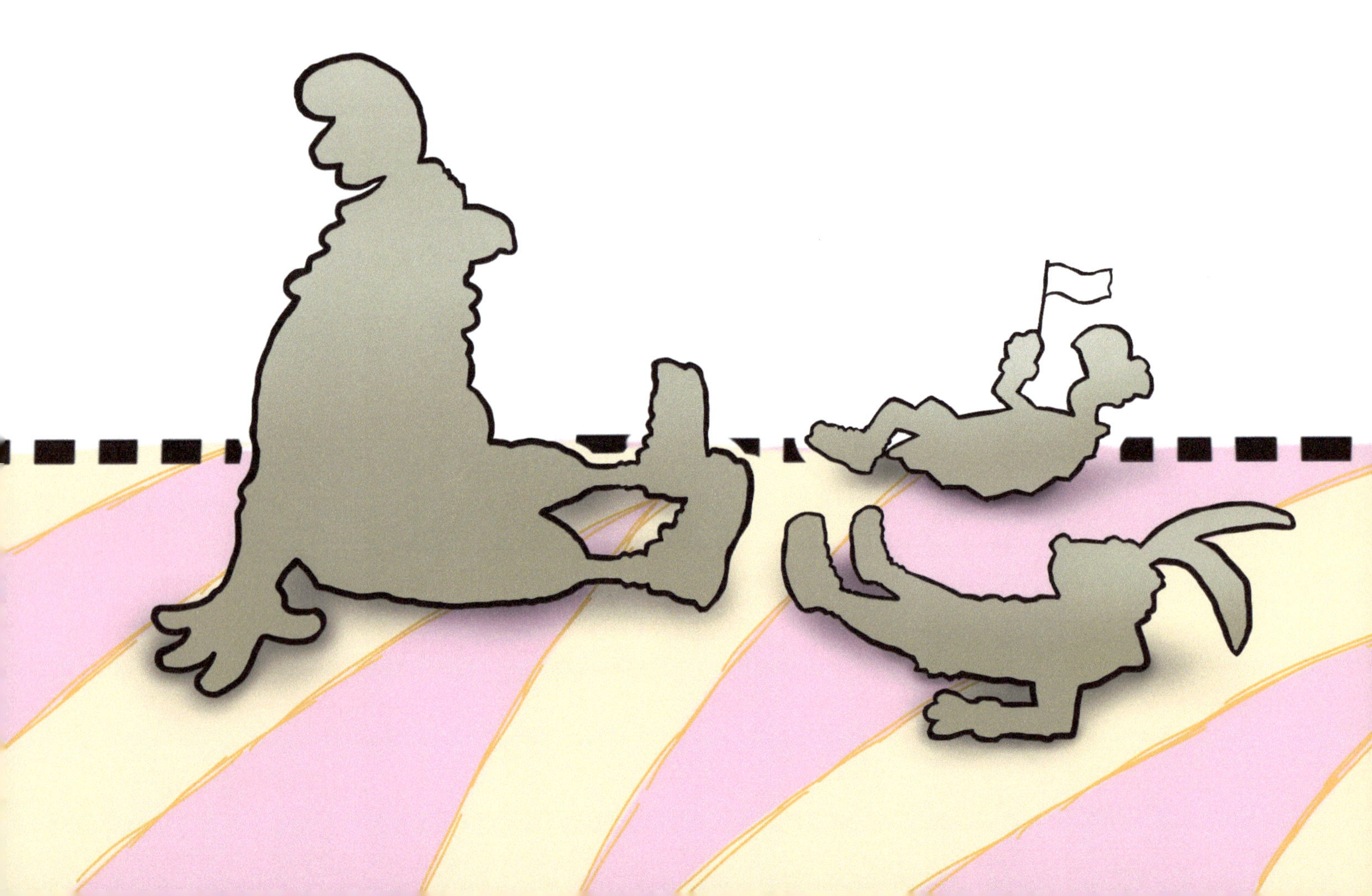

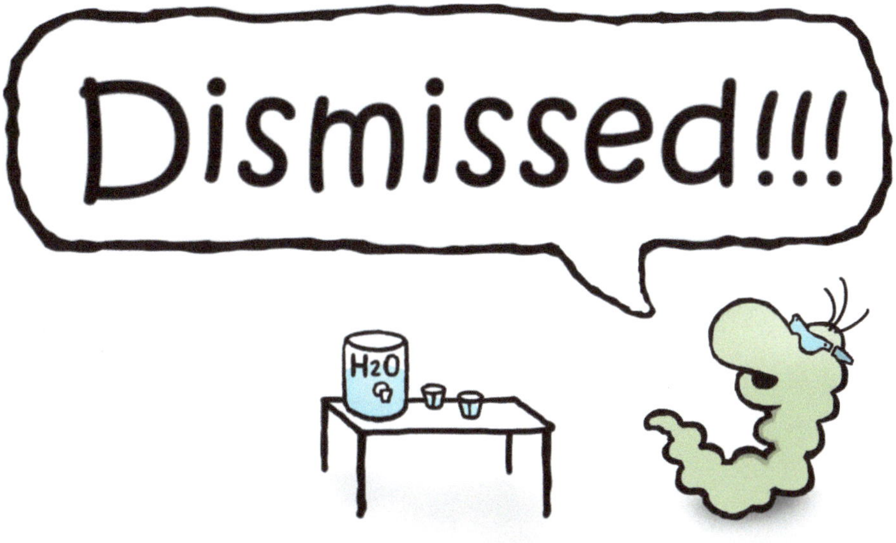

Dismissed!!!
H2O

Chicken Fat Checklist

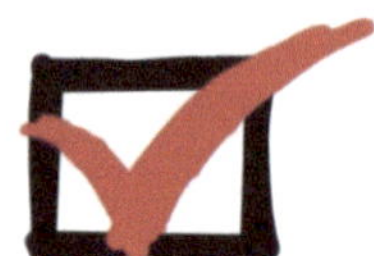

	M	T	W	T	F	S	S
Touch Downs	☐	☐	☐	☐	☐	☐	☐
Push Ups	☐	☐	☐	☐	☐	☐	☐
March In Place	☐	☐	☐	☐	☐	☐	☐
Sit Ups	☐	☐	☐	☐	☐	☐	☐
Twists	☐	☐	☐	☐	☐	☐	☐
Pogo Springs	☐	☐	☐	☐	☐	☐	☐
Jumping Jacks	☐	☐	☐	☐	☐	☐	☐
Arm Circles	☐	☐	☐	☐	☐	☐	☐
Bicycle Ride	☐	☐	☐	☐	☐	☐	☐
Inhale/Exhale	☐	☐	☐	☐	☐	☐	☐
Running In Place	☐	☐	☐	☐	☐	☐	☐

Chicken Fat Checklist

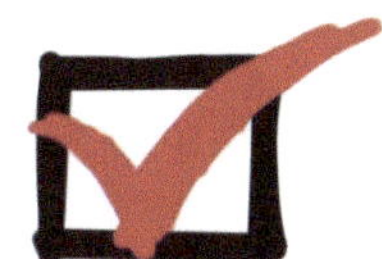

	M	T	W	T	F	S	S
Touch Downs	☐	☐	☐	☐	☐	☐	☐
Push Ups	☐	☐	☐	☐	☐	☐	☐
March In Place	☐	☐	☐	☐	☐	☐	☐
Sit Ups	☐	☐	☐	☐	☐	☐	☐
Twists	☐	☐	☐	☐	☐	☐	☐
Pogo Springs	☐	☐	☐	☐	☐	☐	☐
Jumping Jacks	☐	☐	☐	☐	☐	☐	☐
Arm Circles	☐	☐	☐	☐	☐	☐	☐
Bicycle Ride	☐	☐	☐	☐	☐	☐	☐
Inhale/Exhale	☐	☐	☐	☐	☐	☐	☐
Running In Place	☐	☐	☐	☐	☐	☐	☐

Chicken Fat Checklist 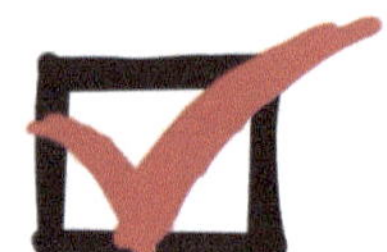

	M	T	W	T	F	S	S
Touch Downs	☐	☐	☐	☐	☐	☐	☐
Push Ups	☐	☐	☐	☐	☐	☐	☐
March In Place	☐	☐	☐	☐	☐	☐	☐
Sit Ups	☐	☐	☐	☐	☐	☐	☐
Twists	☐	☐	☐	☐	☐	☐	☐
Pogo Springs	☐	☐	☐	☐	☐	☐	☐
Jumping Jacks	☐	☐	☐	☐	☐	☐	☐
Arm Circles	☐	☐	☐	☐	☐	☐	☐
Bicycle Ride	☐	☐	☐	☐	☐	☐	☐
Inhale/Exhale	☐	☐	☐	☐	☐	☐	☐
Running In Place	☐	☐	☐	☐	☐	☐	☐

Chicken Fat Checklist 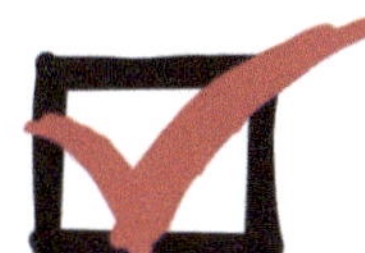

	M	T	W	T	F	S	S
Touch Downs	☐	☐	☐	☐	☐	☐	☐
Push Ups	☐	☐	☐	☐	☐	☐	☐
March In Place	☐	☐	☐	☐	☐	☐	☐
Sit Ups	☐	☐	☐	☐	☐	☐	☐
Twists	☐	☐	☐	☐	☐	☐	☐
Pogo Springs	☐	☐	☐	☐	☐	☐	☐
Jumping Jacks	☐	☐	☐	☐	☐	☐	☐
Arm Circles	☐	☐	☐	☐	☐	☐	☐
Bicycle Ride	☐	☐	☐	☐	☐	☐	☐
Inhale/Exhale	☐	☐	☐	☐	☐	☐	☐
Running In Place	☐	☐	☐	☐	☐	☐	☐

www.ingramcontent.com/pod-product-compliance
Lightning Source LLC
Chambersburg PA
CBHW040201240726
48664CB00002B/787